Cool Plant-Based Recipes

Simple, Healthy Recipes for Living Well

By Frank Rimmel

Sommario

INTRODUCTION

Vegetarianism refers to a lifestyle that excludes the consumption of all forms of meat, including pork, chicken, beef, lamb, venison, fish, and shells.

Depending on a person's beliefs and lifestyle, vegetarianism has different spectrums. There are vegetarians who like to consume products that come from animals such as milk, eggs, cream and cheese. At the other end of the spectrum are vegans.

Vegans never consume meat or any products that come from animals.

The vegan diet has many advantages, in fact, the non-meat intake even following the opinion of many experts can also be a benefit for our body.

In fact, this type of diet is an excellent way to achieve peace between your body and your mind, always remember not to abandon your principles.

Enjoy reading our succulent recipes.

SALADS

Butter Head Lettuce and Triple Cheese Salad

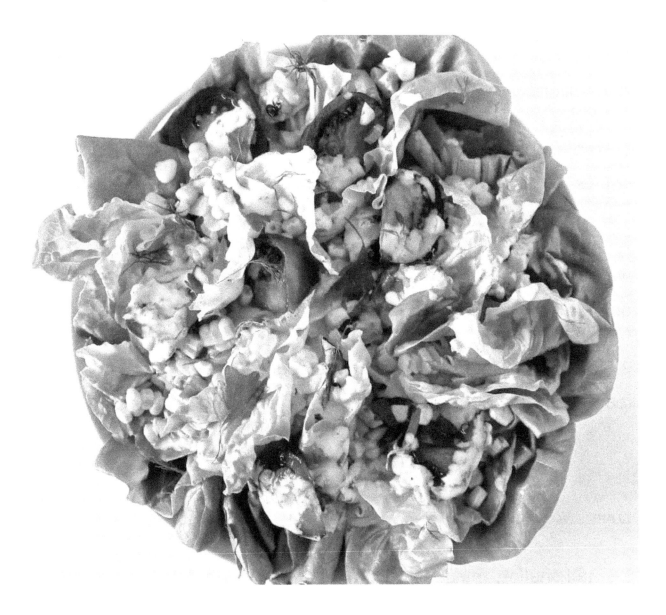

Ingredients:

3 ounces mozarella cheese, shredded

3 ounces pecorino romano cheese, shredded 3 ounces cheddar cheese , shredded

6 cups butter head lettuce, 3 bundles, trimmed

1/4 European or seedless cucumber, halved lengthwise, then thinlysliced

3 tablespoons chopped or snipped chives16 cherry tomatoes

1/2 cup sliced walnuts 1/4 white onion, sliced

2 to 3 tablespoons chopped tarragon leavesSalt and pepper, to taste

Dressing

1 small shallot, minced

1 tablespoon distilled white vinegar
1/4 lemon, juiced, about 2 teaspoons 1/4 cup extra-virgin olive oil

Prep

Combine all of the dressing ingredients in a food processor. Toss with the rest of the ingredients and combine well.

Frisee Lettuce and Two-Cheese Salad

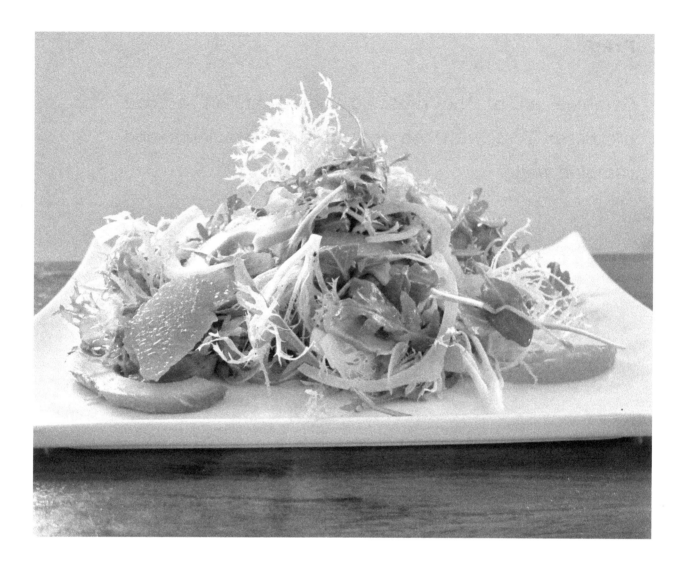

Ingredients:

3 ounces pecorino romano cheese, shredded 3 ounces cheddar cheese , shredded

3 ounces monterey jack cheese, shredded8 ounces vegan cheese

6 to 7 cups frisee lettuce, 3 bundles, trimmed

1/4 European or seedless cucumber, halved lengthwise, then thinlysliced

3 tablespoons chopped or snipped chives16 cherry tomatoes

1/2 cup sliced almonds 1/4 white onion, sliced

2 to 3 tablespoons chopped tarragon leavesSalt and pepper, to taste

Dressing

1 small shallot, minced

1 tablespoon distilled white vinegar
1/4 lemon, juiced, about 2 teaspoons 1/4 cup extra-virgin olive oil

Prep

Combine all of the dressing ingredients in a food processor. Toss with the rest of the ingredients and combine well.

Romaine Lettuce and Tomato Salad

Ingredients:

3 ounces pecorino romano cheese, shredded 3 ounces cheddar cheese , shredded

6 to 7 cups romaine lettuce, 3 bundles, trimmed

1/4 European or seedless cucumber, halved lengthwise, then thinlysliced

3 tablespoons chopped or snipped chives16 cherry tomatoes

1/2 cup sliced cashews 1/4 white onion, sliced

2 to 3 tablespoons chopped rosemary leavesSalt and pepper, to taste

Dressing

1 small shallot, minced

1 tablespoon distilled white vinegar
1/4 lemon, juiced, about 2
teaspoons 1/4 cup extra-virgin
olive oil

Prep

Combine all of the dressing ingredients in a food processor. Toss with the rest of the ingredients and combine well.

Ice Berg Lettuce and Mozarella Salad

Ingredients:

3 ounces mozarella cheese, shredded 3 ounces cheddar cheese , shredded

6 to 7 cups iceberg lettuce, 3 bundles, trimmed

1/4 seedless cucumber, halved lengthwise, then thinly sliced 3 tablespoons chopped or snipped chives

16 small tomatoes 1/2 cup peanuts

1/4 vidalla onion, sliced

2 to 3 tablespoons chopped thyme leaves Salt and pepper, to taste

3 ounces cheddar cheese , shredded

3 ounces monterey jack cheese, shredded

Dressing

1 small shallot, minced

1 tablespoon distilled white vinegar

1/4 lemon, juiced, about 2 teaspoons 1/4 cup extra-virgin olive oil

½ tsp. English mustard

Prep

Combine all of the dressing ingredients in a food processor. Toss with the rest of the ingredients and combine well.

Frisee and Romano Cheese Salad

Ingredients:

7 cups frisee lettuce, 3 bundles, trimmed

1/4 cucumber, halved lengthwise, then thinly sliced3 tablespoons chopped or snipped chives

16 cherry tomatoes

1/2 cup chopped walnuts 1/4 white onion, sliced

2 to 3 tablespoons chopped tarragon leavesSalt and pepper, to taste

3 ounces pecorino romano cheese, shredded 3 ounces cheddar cheese , shredded

3 ounces monterey jack cheese, shredded

Dressing

1 small green onions , minced

1 tablespoon distilled white vinegar

1/4 lemon, juiced, about 2 teaspoons 1/4 cup extra-virgin olive oil

Prep

Combine all of the dressing ingredients in a food processor. Toss with the rest of the ingredients and combine well.

Boston Lettuce and Ricotta Salad

Ingredients:

6 to 7 cups Boston lettuce, 3 bundles, trimmed

1/4 European or seedless cucumber, halved lengthwise, then thinly sliced

3 tablespoons chopped or snipped chives16 cherry tomatoes

1/2 cup sliced walnuts 1/4 red onion, sliced

2 to 3 tablespoons chopped tarragon leavesSalt and pepper, to taste

3 ounces pepperjack cheese, shredded3 ounces ricotta cheese

3 ounces cream cheese, crumbled

Dressing

1 small shallot, minced

1 tablespoon distilled white vinegar
1/4 lemon, juiced, about 2 teaspoons 1/4 cup extra-virgin olive oil

1 tbsp. egg-free mayonnaise

Prep

Combine all of the dressing ingredients in a food processor. Toss with the rest of the ingredients and combine well.

Romaine Lettuce Cherry Tomatoes and Ricotta

Ingredients:

6 to 7 cups Romaine lettuce, 3 bundles, trimmed

1/4 European or seedless cucumber, halved lengthwise, then thinlysliced

3 tablespoons chopped or snipped chives 16 cherry tomatoes

1/2 cup sliced almonds 1/4 white onion, sliced

2 tsp. Herbs de Provence Salt and pepper, to taste 3 ounces ricotta cheese

3 ounces cream cheese, crumbled

3 ounces parmesan cheese, shredded

Dressing

1 small shallot, minced

1 tablespoon distilled white vinegar
1/4 lemon, juiced, about 2 teaspoons 1/4 cup extra-virgin olive oil

Prep

Combine all of the dressing ingredients in a food processor. Toss with the rest of the ingredients and combine well.

Romaine Lettuce Tomatoes and Cream Cheese Salad

Ingredients:

7 cups Romaine lettuce, 3 bundles, trimmed

1/4 European or seedless cucumber, halved lengthwise, then thinly sliced

3 tablespoons chopped or snipped chives 16 cherry tomatoes

1/2 cup sliced walnuts 1/4 white onion, sliced

2 to 3 tablespoons chopped tarragon leaves Salt and pepper, to taste

3 ounces ricotta cheese

3 ounces cream cheese, crumbled

3 ounces parmesan cheese, shredded

Dressing

1 small shallot, minced

1 tablespoon distilled white vinegar
1/4 lemon, juiced, about 2 teaspoons 1/4 cup extra-virgin olive oil

Egg-free mayonnaise

Prep

Combine all of the dressing ingredients in a food processor. Toss with the rest of the ingredients and combine well.

Frisee Lettuce Tomato and Monterey Jack Cheese Salad

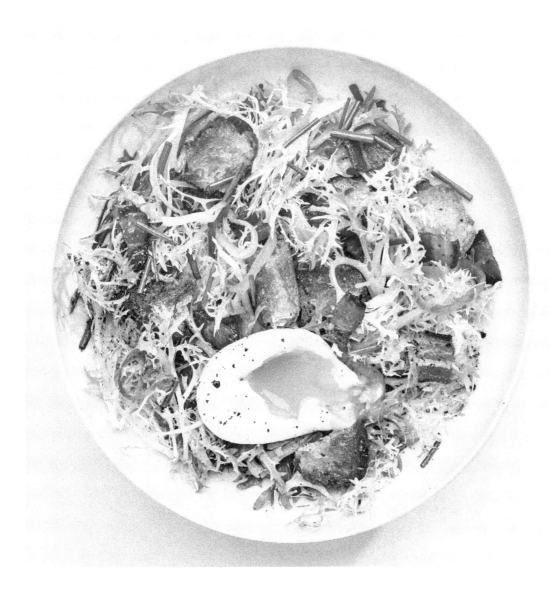

Ingredients:

6 cups Frisee lettuce, 3 bundles, trimmed

1/4 European or seedless cucumber, halved lengthwise, then thinlysliced

3 tablespoons chopped or snipped

chives16 cherry tomatoes

1/2 cup sliced almonds 1/4 red onion, sliced

2 to 3 tablespoons chopped tarragon leavesSalt and pepper, to taste

3 ounces cheddar cheese , shredded

3 ounces monterey jack cheese, shredded3 ounces pepperjack cheese,

Dressing

1 small shallot, minced

1 tablespoon distilled white vinegar 1/4 lemon, juiced, about 2 teaspoons 1/4 cup extra-virgin olive oil

1 tsp. Dijon mustard

Prep

Combine all of the dressing ingredients in a food processor. Toss with the rest of the ingredients and combine well.

Stem Lettuce Cucumber and Parmesan Salad

Ingredients:

6 to 7 cups stem lettuce, 3 bundles, trimmed

1/4 cucumber, halved lengthwise, then thinly sliced 3 tablespoons chopped or snipped chives

2 mangoes, cubed

1/2 cup sliced almonds 1/4 white onion, sliced

2 to 3 tablespoons chopped tarragon leaves Salt and pepper, to taste

6 ounces cream cheese, crumbled

3 ounces parmesan cheese, shredded

Dressing

1 small shallot, minced

1 tablespoon distilled white vinegar1/4 lime, juiced, about 2 teaspoons 1/4 cup extra-virgin olive oil

1 tbsp. honey

1 tsp. English mustard

Prep

Combine all of the dressing ingredients in a food processor. Toss with the rest of the ingredients and combine well.

Stem Lettuce Cherry Tomatoes and Cheddar Cheese Salad

Ingredients:

7 cups stem lettuce, 3 bundles, trimmed

1/4 European or seedless cucumber, halved lengthwise, then thinlysliced

3 tablespoons chopped or snipped chives16 cherry tomatoes

1/2 cup macadamia nuts 1/4 red onion, sliced

2 to 3 tablespoons fresh thyme Salt and pepper, to taste

3 ounces cheddar cheese , shredded

3 ounces monterey jack cheese, shredded

Dressing

1 small shallot, minced

1 tablespoon distilled white vinegar

1/4 lemon, juiced, about 2 teaspoons 1/4 cup extra-virgin olive oil

1 tbsp. honey

1 tsp. Dijon Mustard

Prep

Combine all of the dressing ingredients in a food processor. Toss with the rest of the ingredients and combine well.

Butter head Lettuce Cherry Tomatoes and Pepperjack Cheese Salad

Ingredients:

7 cups iceberg lettuce, 3 bundles, trimmed

1/4 European or seedless cucumber, halved lengthwise, then thinly sliced

3 tablespoons chopped or snipped chives 15 cherry tomatoes

1/2 cup cashews

1/4 white onion, sliced

2 to 3 tablespoons chopped tarragon leaves Salt and pepper, to taste

4 ounces cheddar cheese , shredded 3 ounces pepperjack cheese,

Dressing

1 small shallot, minced

1 tablespoon distilled white vinegar
1/4 lemon, juiced, about 2 teaspoons 1/4 cup extra-virgin olive oil

Prep

Combine all of the dressing ingredients in a food processor. Toss with the rest of the ingredients and combine well.

Romaine Lettuce Cherry Tomatoes and Pecorino Romano Salad

Ingredients:

6 ½ cups Bib lettuce, 3 bundles, trimmed

1/4 European or seedless cucumber, halved lengthwise, then thinlysliced

3 tablespoons chopped or snipped chives16 cherry tomatoes

1/2 cup macadamia nuts 1/4 white onion, sliced

2 to 3 tablespoons chopped tarragon leavesSalt and pepper, to taste

5 ounces pecorino romano cheese, shredded 3 ounces cheddar cheese , shredded

Dressing

1 small shallot, minced

1 tablespoon distilled white vinegar
1/4 lemon, juiced, about 2 teaspoons 1/4 cup extra-virgin olive oil

Prep

Combine all of the dressing ingredients in a food processor. Toss with the rest of the ingredients and combine well.

Iceberg Lettuce Apples and Mozarella Salad

Ingredients:

3 ounces mozarella cheese, shredded 3 ounces cheddar cheese , shredded

3 ounces pepperjack cheese, shredded

6 to 7 cups iceberg lettuce, 3 bundles, trimmed

1/4 European or seedless cucumber, halved lengthwise, then thinly sliced

3 tablespoons chopped or snipped chives

2 apples, cored and cubed into 2 inch cubes 1/2 cup sliced walnuts

1/4 white onion, sliced

2 to 3 tablespoons chopped tarragon leaves Salt and pepper, to taste

Dressing

1 small shallot, minced

2 tablespoons distilled white vinegar1/4 cup sesame oil

1 teaspoon honey

½ tsp. egg-free mayonnaise

Prep

Combine all of the dressing ingredients in a food processor. Toss with the rest of the ingredients and combine well.

Loose-leaf Lettuce Tomatoes and Ricotta Salad

Ingredients:

3 ounces cheddar cheese , shredded

3 ounces pepperjack cheese, shredded3 ounces ricotta cheese

7 cups loose leaf lettuce, 3 bundles, trimmed

1/4 European or seedless cucumber, halved lengthwise, then thinlysliced

3 tablespoons chopped or snipped chives16 cherry tomatoes

1/2 cup sliced almonds 1/4 red onion, sliced

2 to 3 tablespoons chopped thymeSalt and pepper, to taste

Dressing

1 small shallot, minced

1 tablespoon distilled white vinegar
1/4 lemon, juiced, about 2 teaspoons 1/4 cup extra-virgin olive oil

1 tbsp. egg free mayonnaise

Prep

Combine all of the dressing ingredients in a food processor. Toss with the rest of the ingredients and combine well.

Frisee Cherries and Parmesan Salad

Ingredients:

6 to 7 cups frisee lettuce, 3 bundles, trimmed

1/4 European or seedless cucumber, halved lengthwise, then thinly sliced

3 tablespoons chopped or snipped chives 16 cherries, pitted

1/2 cup macadamia nuts 1/4 red onion, sliced

2 to 3 tablespoons chopped tarragon leaves Sea salt and pepper, to taste

3 ounces pepperjack cheese, shredded 3 ounces ricotta cheese

3 ounces parmesan cheese, shredded

Dressing

1 tbsp. chives, snipped

1 tablespoon distilled white vinegar

1/4 lemon, juiced, about 2 teaspoons 1/4 cup extra-virgin olive oil

1 tbsp. honey

Prep

Combine all of the dressing ingredients in a food processor. Toss with the rest of the ingredients and combine well.

Bib Lettuce Grapes and Walnut Salad

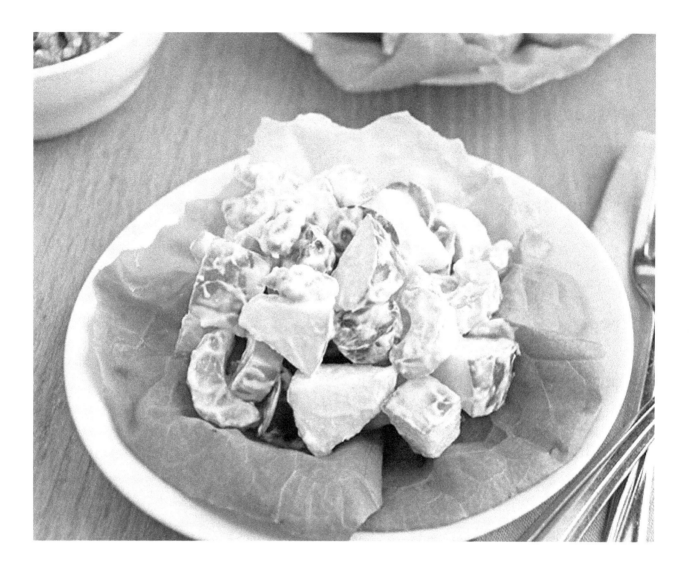

Ingredients:

7 loose bib lettuce, 3 bundles, trimmed

1/4 cucumber, halved lengthwise, then thinly sliced4 tablespoons chopped or snipped chives

16 grapes

1/2 cup sliced walnuts

1/4 white onion, sliced

Salt and pepper, to taste

Dressing

2 tablespoons distilled white vinegar1/4 cup sesame oil

1 tsp. hoi sin sauce

Prep

Combine all of the dressing ingredients in a food processor. Toss with the rest of the ingredients and combine well.

Romaine Lettuce Cherry Tomatoes and Thai Basil Salad

Ingredients:

6 to 7 cups Romaine lettuce, 3 bundles, trimmed

1/4 European or seedless cucumber, halved lengthwise, then thinlysliced

3 tablespoons chopped or snipped chives16 cherry tomatoes

1/2 cup walnuts

1/4 white onion, sliced

2 to 3 tablespoons chopped Thai basilSalt and pepper, to taste

Dressing

1 small scallions, minced

1 tablespoon distilled white vinegar1/4 cup sesame oil

1 tbsp. sambal oelek

Prep

Combine all of the dressing ingredients in a food processor. Toss with the rest of the ingredients and combine well.

Smoky Butter Lettuce and Tarragon Salad

Ingredients:

8 ounces vegan cheese

6 to 7 cups Butter lettuce, 3 bundles, trimmed

1/4 European or seedless cucumber, halved lengthwise, then thinlysliced

3 tablespoons chopped or snipped chives16 cherry tomatoes

1/2 cup sliced almonds 1/4 white onion, sliced

2 to 3 tablespoons chopped tarragon leavesSalt and pepper, to taste

Dressing

1 tsp. cumin

1 tsp. annatto seeds

1 /2 tsp. cayenne pepper

1 tablespoon distilled white vinegar1/4 lime, juiced, about 2 teaspoons 1/4 cup extra-virgin olive oil

Prep

Combine all of the dressing ingredients in a food processor. Toss with the rest of the ingredients and combine well.

Loose-leaf Lettuce Mint Leaves and Cashew Salad

Ingredients:

6 to 7 cups loose leaf lettuce, 3 bundles, trimmed

1/4 European or seedless cucumber, halved lengthwise, then thinly sliced

3 tablespoons chopped or snipped chives 16 grapes

1/2 cup cashews
1/4 red onion, sliced

2 to 3 tablespoons chopped mint leaves Salt and pepper, to taste

3 ounces pepperjack cheese, shredded 3 ounces ricotta cheese

3 ounces parmesan cheese, shredded

Dressing

1 small shallot, minced

1 tablespoon distilled white vinegar1/4 lime, juiced, about 2 teaspoons 1/4 cup extra-virgin olive oil

1 tsp. honey

Prep

Combine all of the dressing ingredients in a food processor. Toss with the rest of the ingredients and combine well.

Romaine Lettuce Tomatoes and Ricotta Salad

Ingredients:

6 to 7 cups romaine lettuce, 3 bundles, trimmed

1/4 European or seedless cucumber, halved lengthwise, then thinlysliced

3 tablespoons chopped or snipped chives16 cherry tomatoes

1/2 cup sliced peanuts
1/4 yellow onion, sliced
Salt and pepper, to
taste 3 ounces ricotta
cheese

3 ounces parmesan cheese, shredded

3 ounces pecorino romano cheese, shredded

Dressing

1 small shallot, minced

1 tablespoon distilled white vinegar

1/4 lemon, juiced, about 2 teaspoons 1/4 cup extra-virgin olive oil

Prep

Combine all of the dressing ingredients in a food processor. Toss with the rest of the ingredients and combine well.

Butter head Lettuce Orange and Monterey Jack Cheese Salad

Ingredients:

6 to 7 cups Butter head lettuce, 3 bundles, trimmed 1/4 cucumber, halved lengthwise, then thinly sliced 3 tablespoons chopped or snipped mint leaves

8 slices of mandarin oranges, skins removed and sliced in half 1/2 cup sliced almonds

1/4 white onion, sliced
Salt and pepper, to taste

3 ounces pecorino romano cheese, shredded 3 ounces cream cheese, crumbled

3 ounces monterey jack cheese, shredded

Dressing

1 small shallot, minced

1 tablespoon distilled white vinegar1/4 lime, juiced, about 2 teaspoons1/4 cup sesame oil

1 tbsp. honey

Prep

Combine all of the dressing ingredients in a food processor. Toss with the rest of the ingredients and combine well.

Simple Lettuce Tomatoes and Pecorino Romano Salad

Ingredients:

6 to 7 cups Romaine lettuce, 3 bundles, trimmed

1/4 European or seedless cucumber, halved lengthwise, then thinlysliced

3 tablespoons chopped or snipped chives16 cherry tomatoes

1/2 cup sliced almonds 1/4 red onion, sliced

2 sprigs of fresh rosemary Salt and pepper, to taste

3 ounces pecorino romano cheese, shredded3 ounces cream cheese, crumbled

3 ounces monterey jack cheese, shredded

Dressing

1 small scallions, minced

1 tablespoon distilled white vinegar

1/4 lemon, juiced, about 2 teaspoons 1/4 cup extra-virgin olive oil

1 egg-free mayonnaise

Prep

Combine all of the dressing ingredients in a food processor. Toss with the rest of the ingredients and combine well.

Romaine Lettuce Tomatoes & Pecorino Romano Salad

Ingredients:

6 to 7 cups Iceberg lettuce, 3 bundles, trimmed

1/4 European or seedless cucumber, halved lengthwise, then thinly sliced

3 tablespoons chopped or snipped chives 16 cherry tomatoes

1/2 cup hazelnuts

10 black grapes, seedless

2 to 3 tablespoons chopped tarragon leaves Salt and pepper, to taste

6 ounces ricotta cheese

1 ounces parmesan cheese, shredded

1 ounces pecorino romano cheese, shredded

Dressing

1 small shallot, minced

1 tablespoon distilled white vinegar

1/4 lemon, juiced, about 2 teaspoons 1/4 cup extra-virgin olive oil

1 tbsp. honey

Prep

Combine all of the dressing ingredients in a food processor. Toss with the rest of the ingredients and combine well.

Butter Lettuce Onion and Tarragon Salad

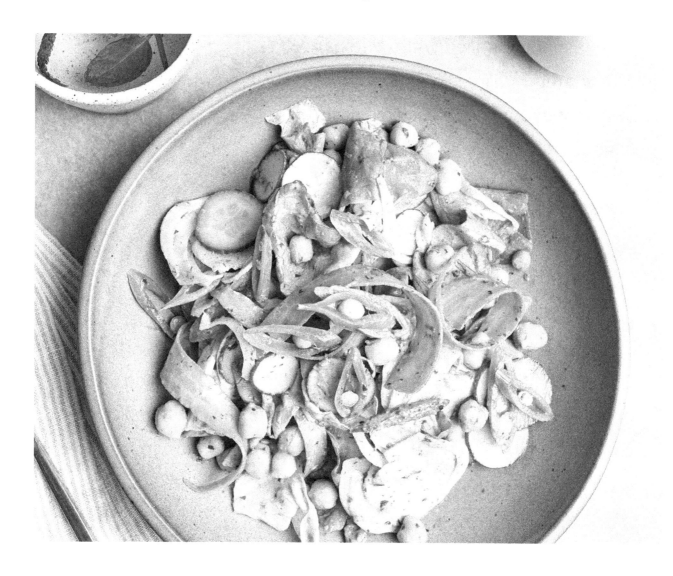

Ingredients:

3 ounces cream cheese, crumbled

3 ounces mozarella cheese, shredded 3 ounces parmesan cheese, shredded

6 to 7 cups Butter lettuce, 3 bundles, trimmed

1/4 European or seedless cucumber, halved lengthwise, then thinly sliced

3 tablespoons chopped or snipped chives16 cherry tomatoes

1/2 cup sliced almonds 1/4 white onion, sliced

2 to 3 tablespoons chopped tarragon leavesSalt and pepper, to taste

Dressing

1 small shallot, minced

1 tablespoon distilled white vinegar
1/4 lemon, juiced, about 2 teaspoons 1/4 cup extra-virgin olive oil

Prep

Combine all of the dressing ingredients in a food

processor. Toss with the rest of the ingredients and combine well.

Romaine Lettuce Tomatoes Almond and Tarragon Salad

Ingredients:

3 ounces pecorino romano cheese, shredded3 ounces cream cheese, crumbled

3 ounces mozarella cheese, shredded

6 to 7 cups Romaine lettuce, 3 bundles, trimmed

1/4 European or seedless cucumber, halved lengthwise, then thinlysliced

3 tablespoons chopped or snipped chives16 cherry tomatoes

1/2 cup sliced almonds 1/4 white onion, sliced

2 to 3 tablespoons chopped tarragon leavesSalt and pepper, to taste

Dressing

1 small shallot, minced

1 tablespoon distilled white vinegar

1/4 lemon, juiced, about 2 teaspoons 1/4 cup extra-virgin olive oil

Prep

Combine all of the dressing ingredients in a food processor. Toss with the rest of the ingredients and combine well.

Romaine Tomatoes with Cream Cheese and Hazelnut Salad

Ingredients:

3 ounces monterey jack cheese, shredded 3 ounces ricotta cheese

3 ounces cheddar cheese , shredded

6 to 7 cups Romaine lettuce, 3 bundles, trimmed

1/4 European or seedless cucumber, halved lengthwise, then thinly sliced

3 tablespoons chopped or snipped chives 16 cherry tomatoes

1/2 cup sliced hazelnuts 1/4 white onion, sliced

2 to 3 tablespoons chopped tarragon leaves Salt and pepper, to taste

Dressing

1 small shallot, minced

1 tablespoon distilled white vinegar
1/4 lemon, juiced, about 2 teaspoons 1/4 cup extra-virgin olive oil

Prep

Combine all of the dressing ingredients in a food processor. Toss with the rest of the ingredients and combine well.

Butter Lettuce and Zucchini with Parmesan Salad

Ingredients:

5 ounces cream cheese, crumbled

3 ounces mozarella cheese, shredded 1 ounces parmesan cheese, shredded

6 to 7 cups Butter lettuce, 3 bundles, trimmed

1/4 Zucchini, halved lengthwise, then thinly sliced 16 cherry tomatoes

1/2 cup sliced almonds 1/4 white onion, sliced

2 to 3 tablespoons chopped tarragon leavesSalt and pepper, to taste

Dressing

1 small shallot, minced

1 tablespoon distilled white vinegar

1/4 lemon, juiced, about 2 teaspoons 1/4 cup extra-virgin olive oil

Prep

Combine all of the dressing ingredients in a food processor. Toss with the rest of the ingredients and combine well.

Romaine Lettuce with Mozarella and Hazelnut Salad

Ingredients:

6 ounces mozarella cheese, shredded 3 ounces parmesan cheese, shredded

6 to 7 cups Romaine lettuce, 3 bundles, trimmed

1/4 European or seedless cucumber, halved lengthwise, then thinly sliced

3 tablespoons chopped or snipped chives16 cherry tomatoes

1/2 cup sliced hazelnuts 1/4 white onion, sliced

2 to 3 tablespoons chopped tarragon leavesSalt and pepper, to taste

Dressing

1 small shallot, minced

1 tablespoon distilled white vinegar
1/4 lemon, juiced, about 2 teaspoons 1/4 cup extra-virgin olive oil

Prep

Combine all of the dressing ingredients in a food processor. Toss with the rest of the ingredients and combine well.

Iceberg Lettuce Tomatoes Mozarella and Almond Salad

Ingredients:

3 ounces cream cheese, crumbled

5 ounces mozarella cheese, shredded

6 to 7 cups Iceberg lettuce, 3 bundles, trimmed

1/4 European or seedless cucumber, halved lengthwise, then thinlysliced

3 tablespoons chopped or snipped chives16 cherry tomatoes

1/2 cup sliced almonds 1/4 white onion, sliced

2 to 3 tablespoons chopped tarragon leavesSalt and pepper, to taste

Dressing

1 small shallot, minced

1 tablespoon distilled white vinegar

1/4 lemon, juiced, about 2 teaspoons 1/4 cup extra-virgin olive oil

Prep

Combine all of the dressing ingredients in a food processor. Toss with the rest of the ingredients and combine well.

Romaine Lettuce Cream Cheese and Pistachio Salad

Ingredients:

5 ounces cream cheese, crumbled

3 ounces mozarella cheese, shredded

6 to 7 cups Romaine lettuce, 3 bundles, trimmed

1/4 European or seedless cucumber, halved lengthwise, then thinly sliced

3 tablespoons chopped or snipped chives 16 cherry tomatoes

1/2 cup sliced pistachios 1/4 Vidalla onion, sliced

2 to 3 tablespoons chopped tarragon leaves Salt and pepper, to taste

Dressing

1 small shallot, minced

1 tablespoon distilled white vinegar

1/4 lemon, juiced, about 2 teaspoons 1/4 cup extra-virgin olive oil

Prep

Combine all of the dressing ingredients in a food processor. Toss with the rest of the ingredients and combine well.

Frisee Mozarella and Feta Salad

Ingredients:

6 to 7 cups butter head lettuce, 3 bundles, trimmed

1/4 seedless cucumber, halved lengthwise, then thinly sliced 3 tablespoons chopped or snipped chives

16 cherry tomatoes 1/2 cup pistachios

1/4 white onion, sliced

2 to 3 tablespoons chopped tarragon leaves Salt and pepper, to taste

3 ounces mozarella cheese, shredded 6 ounces parmesan cheese, shredded

Dressing

1 small shallot, minced

1 tablespoon distilled white vinegar

1/4 lemon, juiced, about 2 teaspoons 1/4 cup extra-virgin olive oil

1 tbsp. pesto sauce

Prep

Combine all of the dressing ingredients in a food processor. Toss with the rest of the ingredients and combine well.

Romaine Lettuce with Pepperjack and Feta Salad

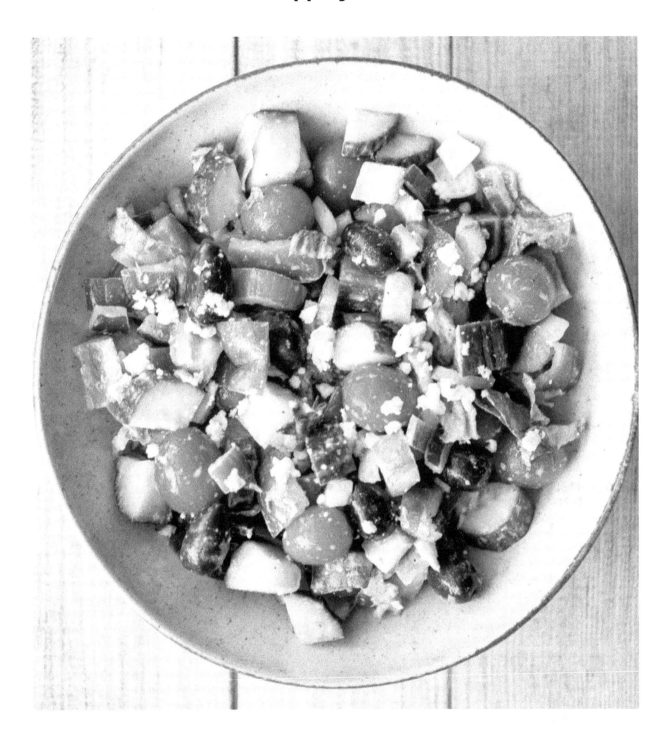

Ingredients:

6 to 7 cups romaine lettuce, 3 bundles, trimmed

1/4 European or seedless cucumber, halved lengthwise, then thinly sliced

3 tablespoons chopped or snipped chives 16 cherry tomatoes

1/2 cup macadamia nuts 1/4 red onion, sliced Salt and pepper, to taste

1 ounces monterey jack cheese, shredded 3 ounces ricotta cheese

1 ounces cheddar cheese , shredded

1 ounces pepperjack cheese, shredded

Dressing

1 small shallot, minced

1 tablespoon distilled white vinegar 1/4 lemon, juiced, about 2 teaspoons 1/4 cup extra-virgin olive oil

1 tbsp. pesto sauce

Prep

Combine all of the dressing ingredients in a food processor. Toss with the rest of the ingredients and combine well.

Loose-leaf Lettuce Tomato and 4 Cheese Salad

Ingredients:

6 to 7 cups loose leaf lettuce, 3 bundles, trimmed 1/4 cucumber, halved lengthwise, then thinly sliced 16 cherry tomatoes

1/4 red onion, sliced

2 to 3 tablespoons chopped fresh basil Salt and pepper, to taste

2 ounces cheddar cheese , shredded

2 ounces pepperjack cheese, shredded

3 ounces pecorino romano cheese, shredded 2 ounces cream cheese, crumbled

Dressing

1 small shallot, minced

1 tablespoon distilled white vinegar
1/4 lemon, juiced, about 2

teaspoons 1/4 cup extra-virgin olive oil

Prep

Combine all of the dressing ingredients in a food processor. Toss with the rest of the ingredients and combine well.

Frisee Lettuce Tomatoes and Pecorino Romano

Ingredients:

6 to 7 cups frisee lettuce, 3 bundles, trimmed

1/4 cucumber, halved lengthwise, then thinly sliced 3 tablespoons chopped or snipped chives

16 cherry tomatoes
1/2 cup sliced
almonds 1/4 red
onion, sliced

2 to 3 tablespoons chopped parsley Salt and pepper, to taste

3 ounces ricotta cheese

2 ounces cheddar cheese , shredded

1 ounces pepperjack cheese, shredded

1 ounces pecorino romano cheese, shredded

Dressing

1 small scallions, minced

1 tablespoon distilled white vinegar

1/4 lemon, juiced, about 2 teaspoons 1/4 cup macadamia nut oil

Prep

Combine all of the dressing ingredients in a food processor. Toss with the rest of the ingredients and combine well.

Romaine Lettuce Tomatoes and Ricotta

Ingredients:

2 ounces monterey jack cheese, shredded 2 ounces ricotta cheese

2 ounces cheddar cheese , shredded

2 ounces pepperjack cheese, shredded

6 to 7 cups romaine lettuce, 3 bundles, trimmed

1/4 European or seedless cucumber, halved lengthwise, then thinly sliced

3 tablespoons chopped or snipped chives 16 cherry tomatoes

1/2 cup pistachios
1/4 red onion, sliced

Salt and pepper, to taste

Dressing

1 small shallot, minced

1 tablespoon distilled white vinegar
1/4 lemon, juiced, about 2 teaspoons 1/4 cup extra-virgin olive oil

Prep

Combine all of the dressing ingredients in a food processor. Toss with the rest of the ingredients and combine well.

Loose-leaf Lettuce and Pecorino Romano Salad

Ingredients:

3 ounces pepperjack cheese, shredded

3 ounces pecorino romano cheese, shredded3 ounces cream cheese, crumbled

3 ounces mozarella cheese, shredded

6 to 7 cups loose leaf head lettuce, 3 bundles, trimmed 1/4 cucumber, halved lengthwise, then thinly sliced

3 tablespoons snipped chives16 cherry tomatoes

1/2 cup peanuts

1/4 white onion, sliced
Salt and pepper, to taste

Dressing

1 small shallot, minced

2 tablespoon distilled white vinegar1/4 cup sesame seed oil

1 tbsp. Thai chili garlic sauce

Prep

Combine all of the dressing ingredients in a food processor. Toss with the rest of the ingredients and combine well.

Butterhead Chives and Pistachio Salad

Ingredients:

7 cups loose butterhead lettuce, 3 bundles, trimmed

1/4 European or seedless cucumber, halved lengthwise, then thinlysliced

3 tablespoons chopped or snipped chives16 grapes

1/2 cup pistachios 1/4 onion, sliced

Salt and pepper, to taste 6 ounces vegan cheese

Dressing

1 sprig parsley, chopped

1 tablespoon distilled white vinegar

1/4 lemon, juiced, about 2 teaspoons 1/4 cup extra-virgin olive oil

Prep

Combine all of the dressing ingredients in a food processor. Toss with the rest of the ingredients and combine well.

Boston Lettuce Almond and Vegan Cream Cheese Salad

Ingredients:

7 cups Boston lettuce, 3 bundles, trimmed

½ cucumber, halved lengthwise, then thinly sliced 3 tablespoons chopped or snipped chives

16 cherry tomatoes
1/2 cup sliced
almonds 1/4 red
onion, sliced

Salt and pepper, to taste

7 ounces vegan cream cheese

Dressing

1 small shallot, minced

1 tablespoon distilled white vinegar
1/4 lemon, juiced, about 2
teaspoons 1/4 cup extra-virgin

olive oil

1 tbsp. chimichurri sauce

Prep

Combine all of the dressing ingredients in a food processor. Toss with the rest of the ingredients and combine well.

Frisee Lettuce and Tomato Salad d

Ingredients:

6 to 7 cups Frisee lettuce, 3 bundles, trimmed

1/4 cucumber, halved lengthwise, then thinly sliced3 tablespoons chopped or snipped chives

16 cherry tomatoes
1/2 cup sliced
almonds 1/4 red
onion, sliced

Salt and pepper, to taste

3 ounces pepperjack cheese, shredded

3 ounces pecorino romano cheese, shredded3 ounces cream cheese, crumbled

3 ounces mozarella cheese, shredded

Dressing

1 sprig parsley, minced

1 tablespoon distilled white vinegar

1/4 lemon, juiced, about 2 teaspoons 1/4 cup extra-virgin olive oil

Prep

Combine all of the dressing ingredients in a food processor. Toss with the rest of the ingredients and combine well.

Mesclun and Tomato with Cilantro Vinaigrette

Ingredients:

6 to 7 cups mesclun, 3 bundles, trimmed

1/4 cucumber, halved lengthwise, then thinly sliced 3 tablespoons chopped or snipped chives

16 cherry tomatoes
1/2 cup sliced
almonds 1/4 white
onion, sliced

Salt and pepper, to taste

1 ounce blue cheese, crumbled

3 ounces gouda cheese,
shredded 3 ounces brie cheese,
crumbled

Dressing

1 sprig cilantro, minced

1 tablespoon distilled white vinegar

1/4 lemon, juiced, about 2 teaspoons 1/4 cup extra-virgin olive oil

Prep

Combine all of the dressing ingredients in a food processor. Toss with the rest of the ingredients and combine well.

Chervil and Almond Salad

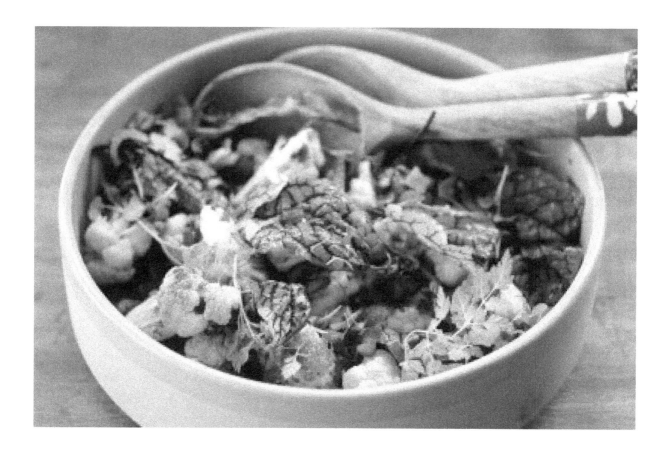

Ingredients:

7 cups chervil, 3 bundles, trimmed

1/4 cucumber, halved lengthwise, then thinly sliced 3 tablespoons chopped or snipped chives

16 cherry tomatoes
1/2 cup sliced
almonds 1/4 white
onion, sliced

Salt and pepper, to taste

3 ounces parmesan cheese, shredded 1 ounce blue cheese, crumbled

3 ounces gouda cheese, shredded

Dressing

1 tablespoon distilled white vinegar
1/4 lemon, juiced, about 2 teaspoons 1/4 cup extra-virgin olive oil

1 tsp. English mustard

Prep

Combine all of the dressing ingredients in a food processor. Toss with the rest of the ingredients and combine well.

Bib Lettuce and Vegan Ricotta Salad

Ingredients:

6 to 7 cups bib lettuce, 3 bundles, trimmed

1/4 cucumber, halved lengthwise, then thinly sliced16 grapes

1/2 cup sliced almonds
1/4 white onion, sliced
Salt and pepper, to
taste

3 ounces mozarella cheese, shredded 3 ounces parmesan cheese, shredded 1 ounce blue cheese, crumbled

Dressing

1 tablespoon distilled white vinegar
1/4 lemon, juiced, about 2 teaspoons 1/4 cup extra-virgin olive oil

1 tbsp. Chimichurri sauce

Prep

Combine all of the dressing ingredients in a food processor. Toss with the rest of the ingredients and combine well.

Boston Lettuce Walnut and Vegan Parmesan Salad

Ingredients:

6 to 7 cups boston lettuce, 3 bundles, trimmed

1/4 cucumber, halved lengthwise, then thinly sliced 3 tablespoons chopped or snipped chives

16 tomatillos, sliced in half 1/2 cup walnuts

1/4 red onion, sliced
Salt and pepper, to taste

3 ounces camembert cheese, crumbled 3 ounces mozarella cheese, shredded 3 ounces parmesan cheese, shredded

Dressing

1 tablespoon distilled white vinegar
1/4 lemon, juiced, about 2

teaspoons 1/4 cup extra-virgin olive oil

1 tsp. egg free mayonnaise

Prep

Combine all of the dressing ingredients in a food processor. Toss with the rest of the ingredients and combine well.

Endive Lettuce Tomatillo and Vegan Ricotta Salad

Ingredients:

6 to 7 cups endive, 3 bundles, trimmed

1/4 cucumber, halved lengthwise, then thinly sliced3 tablespoons chopped or snipped chives

16 green tomatillos, sliced in half1/2 cup sliced almonds

1/4 white onion, sliced
Salt and pepper, to
taste

3 ounces pecorino romano cheese, shredded3 ounces cream cheese, crumbled

3 ounces camembert cheese, crumbled

Dressing

1 tablespoon distilled white vinegar
1/4 lemon, juiced, about 2

teaspoons 1/4 cup extra-virgin olive oil

1 tsp. Dijon mustard

Prep

Combine all of the dressing ingredients in a food processor. Toss with the rest of the ingredients and combine well.

Kale Tomato and Vegan Parmesan Salad

Ingredients:

6 to 7 cups kale, 3 bundles, trimmed

1/4 cucumber, halved lengthwise, then thinly sliced3 tablespoons chopped or snipped chives

16 cherry tomatoes
1/2 cup sliced
almonds 1/4 white
onion, sliced

Salt and pepper, to taste

3 ounces pepperjack cheese, shredded

3 ounces pecorino romano cheese, shredded3 ounces cream cheese, crumbled

Dressing

1 sprig cilantro, minced

1 tablespoon distilled white vinegar

1/4 lemon, juiced, about 2 teaspoons 1/4 cup extra-virgin olive oil

1 tsp. egg free mayonnaise

Prep

Combine all of the dressing ingredients in a food processor. Toss with the rest of the ingredients and combine well.

Lettuce Tomatillos and Almond Salad

Ingredients:

6 to 7 cups lettuce, 3 bundles, trimmed

1/4 cucumber, halved lengthwise, then thinly sliced 3 tablespoons chopped or snipped chives

16 tomatillos, sliced in half 1/2 cup sliced almonds 1/4 white onion, sliced Salt and pepper, to taste

3 ounces cream cheese, crumbled

3 ounces camembert cheese, crumbled 3 ounces mozarella cheese, shredded

Dressing

1 sprig cilantro, minced

1 tablespoon distilled white vinegar

1/4 lemon, juiced, about 2 teaspoons 1/4 cup extra-virgin olive oil

1 tsp. English mustard

Prep

Combine all of the dressing ingredients in a food processor. Toss with the rest of the ingredients and combine well.

Kale Tomato and Almond Salad

Ingredients:

6 to 7 cups kale, 3 bundles, trimmed

1/4 cucumber, halved lengthwise, then thinly sliced 3 tablespoons chopped or snipped chives

16 cherry tomatoes
1/2 cup sliced
almonds 1/4 white
onion, sliced

Salt and pepper, to taste

3 ounces camembert cheese, crumbled 3 ounces mozarella cheese, shredded 3 ounces parmesan cheese, shredded

Dressing

1 sprig cilantro, minced

1 tablespoon distilled white vinegar

1/4 lemon, juiced, about 2 teaspoons 1/4 cup extra-virgin olive oil

1 tsp. English mustard

Prep

Combine all of the dressing ingredients in a food processor. Toss with the rest of the ingredients and combine well.

Kale Almond and Vegan Ricotta Salad

Ingredients:

6 to 7 cups kale, 3 bundles, trimmed

1/4 cucumber, halved lengthwise, then thinly sliced 3 tablespoons chopped or snipped chives

16 green tomatillos, sliced in half 1/2 cup sliced almonds

1/4 white onion, sliced
Salt and pepper, to taste

3 ounces cottage cheese, crumbled

3 ounces pepperjack cheese, shredded

3 ounces pecorino romano cheese, shredded

Dressing

1 tablespoon distilled white vinegar
1/4 lemon, juiced, about 2

teaspoons 1/4 cup extra-virgin olive oil

1 tsp. Dijon mustard

Prep

Combine all of the dressing ingredients in a food processor. Toss with the rest of the ingredients and combine well.

Conclusion

We have reached the end of this fantastic cookbook, Did you and the whole family have fun cooking and preparing these tasty recipes?

I sure hope so.

A perfect combination for maintaining physical and emotional well-being.

I send you a big hug and hope to continue to keep you company with our vegetarian recipes that allow you to not give up taste.

This conclusion is for a family book but can be adapted to anything.

CPSIA information can be obtained
at www.ICGtesting.com
Printed in the USA
LVHW061628180421
684848LV00003B/558